27 |
To Help You Become A
Cigar Expert

The Guide To Learning What You Need To Know About Cigar Smoking Etiquette, Lighting, Cutting, Buying, Spotting Fake Cubans, And Much More

Brought to you by:
CashIsFun.com

DISCLAIMER

This book is intended for information purposes only and is not in any way an endorsement of smoking.

SMOKING HAS BEEN LINKED TO SERIOUS HEALTH PROBLEMS

The content of this book was complied both from publically available sources and the personal knowledge of the author, and is believed to be entirely accurate, though it is *not* guaranteed to be without errors.

Please see pages 45-46 for more health information specific to smoking cigars.

Congratulations!

Congratulations on taking this step into the fun, exciting, sophisticated, interesting, and always entertaining world of cigars. We know you will enjoy this book and learn lots of great information from it.

If you have any questions or comments about the book, we'd love to hear from you by email at:

books@cashisfun.com

April 2010

Index

Introduction 1
#1. Cigar Smoking Basics 3
#2. Cigar Terms 5
#3. History Of Cigars 7
#4. How Cigars Are Made 9
#5. Where To Buy Cigars 11
#6. Sizes And Styles 13
#7. Choosing The Best Single 15
#8. Top Brands 16
#9. Types Of Cutters 17
#10. Making A Perfect Cut 19
#11. Proper Lighting Technique 20
#12. All About Ashing 21
#13. Being A Courteous Smoker 23
#14. Quality Test 25
#15. Pairing With Alcohol 26
#16. Pairing With Food 27
#17. Get A Humidor 28
#18. Vintage And Aged Cigars 29
#19. Don't Break The 70-70 Rule 30
#20. The Cuban Holy Grail 31
#21. Spotting Fake Cubans 33
#22. Give The Gift Of Smoke 35
#23. Blowing Smoke Rings 37
#24. Fighting The Beetles 38
#25. Cigar Bars 40
#26. Cigar-Friendly Activities 41
#27. Parties 43
CashIsFun.com 44
Health Risks 45
Cigar Sites Directory 47
Notes 50

Introduction

Special introduction message to this book and the world of cigars from Fred Rewey:

Cigar smoking is an experience.

From the moment you walk into the cigar store to the final puff, it can be an adventure. It is those in-between moments that can elude us. Where to store them, which cigar to smoke, how to light it, etc, etc.

I remember spending one cold winter day in my garage learning to blow smoke rings. I also remember visiting Key West, lighting a cigar at 10:30 AM outside a general store, and how this very act prompted conversation with a local that could only be characterized properly in a Hemingway novel.

This book, *27 Lessons to Help You Become a Cigar Expert*, which was created by the team at CashIsFun.com, tackles the most common questions in an easy-to-read, easy-to-implement format.

Although the world of cigars can be immense, this book provides a short list of tips that can get you started and informed to the point where you won't be embarrassed to walk into your local smoke shop, grab a cigar, and talk "shop" with another patron.

Cigar smoking envelops its own set of etiquette, procedures, and standards. With that said, do whatever you want. Because, in the end, it is your tastes that matter--not your friends', and not mine.

FREE Digital Copy, Updates, and More Information Available Here:
www.CashIsFun.com/cigar

Consider *27 Lessons to Help You Become a Cigar Expert* a quest to find your true cigar smoking character and this guide a map to help you find your way.

I wish you all the best in your cigar "research" and hope that someday, in the not too distant future, we will meet up in some small cigar shop.

-Fred "The Godfather" Rewey
Founder of CigarSecrets.com
April 5, 2010

FREE Digital Copy, Updates, and More Information Available Here:
www.CashIsFun.com/cigar

#1

Cigar Smoking Basics

First, congratulations for getting this book! Read it carefully and these lessons will teach you everything you need to know to get started with cigar smoking...

Be sure to keep in mind that smoking a cigar is not the same as smoking a cigarette. You smoke a cigar to enjoy the smells and flavors of the smoke. Think of being a cigar expert as similar to being a wine expert. Good cigars and good wines have a lot in common.

Cigars are made with premium quality tobacco. Similar to how the taste of wine has a lot to do with the grapes it is made from and how the wine is taken care of during and after the bottling process, flavors you get from cigars also strongly depend on different factors, such as the quality of the soil used, the type of tobacco, weather conditions, the age of the cigar, and even the type of environment the cigar has been stored in since it was made.

When you smoke a cigar, do not inhale the smoke into your lungs like a cigarette. You draw it carefully into your mouth then blow it out slowly.

FREE Digital Copy, Updates, and More Information Available Here:
www.CashIsFun.com/cigar

The smoke should never reach your lungs, later there will be more information about the health risks involved with cigars.

Do not smoke too quickly. Smoking too quickly will overheat your cigar and "burn" the smoke, altering the flavor. You will only want to take a puff on your cigar every 30-40 seconds, and every 5-6 puffs you'll want to blow a little air through your cigar to clear any smoke out so it does not get stale. A good cigar should take over an hour to smoke.

Lighting and ashing are also different with cigars than with cigarettes, but those issues will also be covered in later lessons.

Just remember to relax and enjoy! A good cigar, especially when paired with the right drink, can be an excellent experience.

FREE Digital Copy, Updates, and More Information Available Here: www.CashIsFun.com/cigar

#2

Cigar Terms

Here are some important cigar terms that every cigar smoker should know:

- Band - The often colorful ring of paper that is close to the closed end of the cigar. After you light the cigar and it heats up a bit, it is usually possible to slide the band off easily.
- Bouquet - The smell of a good cigar, or the "nose." If you do not store your cigars correctly, they will lose their bouquet.
- Box - A set of 25 or 50 premium cigars.
- Bundle - A group of 25 of 50 cigars, usually less expensive and lower quality than boxed cigars.
- Cap - The piece of leaf placed on one end of the cigar to hold the wrapper in place.
- Cedar - The type of wood used in most cigar humidors and boxes. A thin piece of cedar is also wrapped around some premium cigars for lighting.
- Handmade - As opposed to machine rolled. All premium cigars are handmade and used better quality materials.

FREE Digital Copy, Updates, and More Information Available Here:
www.CashIsFun.com/cigar

- Hot - If the tobacco is too loosely packed it can cause the cigar to overheat and alter the flavors.

- Humidor - Any storage area from the size of a small box to an entire room that is designed to keep cigars at the perfect 70°F/70% humidity level.

- Long Filler - Good quality tobacco that runs the entire length of the cigar, as opposed to short filler that is usually used in cheap machine-made cigars.

- Plugged - If the tobacco is too tightly packed it can cause the cigar to burn too slowly or go out too easily.

- Shoulder - Part of the cigar where the wrapper and the cap come together; cut past this and your cigar will probably start to come apart.

- Spill - A small piece of cedar that you can light first, then light your cigar with.

FREE Digital Copy, Updates, and More Information Available Here:
www.CashIsFun.com/cigar

#3

History Of Cigars

Today cigars are produced and enjoyed all over the world, but tobacco is indigenous only to the Americas. Today, most cigars come from Caribbean Sea area nations, such as Jamaica, Dominican Republic, Honduras, Nicaragua, and most famously, Cuba.

By the time the first European explorers started coming to the Americas, the native people had been cultivating and smoking tobacco for many generations. It is believed that the Maya of Yucatan peninsula in modern day Mexico and parts of Central America were the first to cultivate tobacco.

The first tobacco plantations in the United States were established in Virginia and Maryland but at first tobacco was only smoked in pipes.

The cigar was not introduced to the United States until the late 18th century. Israel Putnam, an army general who had served in the Revolutionary War, is credited with introducing the cigar to the United States. He had traveled to Cuba after the Revolutionary War and returned with a box of

Cuban cigars. Their popularity quickly spread after that.

In Europe, cigar production and consumption did not achieve widespread popularity until after the Peninsula War in the early 19th century. British and French veterans returned to their homelands after years of serving in Spain with their tobacco pipes in tow. Among the rich and fashionable, the favored method of taking tobacco was the cigar. Cigar smoking remains a habit associated with the rich and discriminating of upper society.

#4

How Cigars Are Made

1. Sorting - The different types of tobacco are sorted and grouped by such qualities as color, texture, and strength.
2. Blending - Each brand of cigar has it's own special "blend" of tobaccos that gives it its unique flavor.
3. Bunching - The blend is grouped into a cylindrical shape and checked to make sure it is uniform and straight.
4. Binding - The bunch of tobacco is tightly wrapped in a binder layer that gives the cigar its shape, structure, and ability to hold moisture.
5. Molding - The mold contains a group of binded cigars and presses them into their shape so they will be tightly packed.
6. Weight Inspecting - After the mold, finished cigars are put into bundles of 50 and weighed to ensure they were not rolled too loosely or too tightly.

FREE Digital Copy, Updates, and More Information Available Here:
www.CashIsFun.com/cigar

7. Hand Inspecting - After passing the weight test the cigars are inspected by hand for quality of the filler, binder, and wrapper.

8. Storing - The finished cigars are placed in cedar containers and aged for up to a year. This adds flavor, helps to ensure the cigar will burn better, and that all of the cigars have a uniform taste.

9. Coloring - The cigars are then grouped by color so all 25 cigars in a box are the exact same shade.

FREE Digital Copy, Updates, and More Information Available Here:
www.CashIsFun.com/cigar

#5
Where To Buy Cigars

The best place is buy top quality cigars is your local tobacconist shop. The staff should be knowledgeable and helpful so they can answer any questions you may have. They can help you figure out which cigar is best for you. If you need help learning how to light or store or anything else related to your cigar smoking experience, your local tobacconist should be your first stop. You might even get a good story, or some interesting lore out of these guys.

Many liquor stores have started installing humidor rooms and stocking fine cigars of many different brands. If the location or hours of operation are more convenient for you than a true tobacconist, then these liquor stores can be a great alternative place to get your cigars. However, you may find that some of the staff may not be knowledgeable as the people you fill find working at a tobacconist shop.

If you know exactly what you want, the internet is now a great place to buy cigars; often for much less than you can get in the shops. The internet is especially good for finding sample packages of all

FREE Digital Copy, Updates, and More Information Available Here:
www.CashIsFun.com/cigar

different kinds. So especially if you are new to cigar smoking you can get a humidor and start buying sample packs of different brands, and sizes, and types to learn what you really like. Or if you already know what you like, you can buy them in bulk. Check out the directory near the end of this book or sign up at *www.CashIsFun.com/cigar* to get a list of good cigar sites.

#6

Sizes And Styles

All cigars can be divided into two broad categories: parejos and figurados.

Parejos refers to cigars that are basically straight. They are subdivided into three categories: coronas, panatelas, and lonsdales. Coronas come in a variety of styles and famous brands. They are known as cigars with an 'open foot' (or tip) and a rounded head. Panatelas are generally longer than coronas, are thinner. Lonsdales are also longer than coronas, but are thinner than panatelas.

The second basic category consists of the figurados. Figurados refers to cigars with that are irregular or somehow hand-shaped so that they are not strictly straight. The smallest type of figurados is the belicoso cigars, which are known for a larger foot and a smaller, rounded head. Another basic figurado cigar is the pyramid, which have pointed heads that taper to a large foot. The perfecto is a figurado cigar that is tapered on both the head and foot, with a thinner middle. The largest figurado is the diademas, known as the 'giant' of cigars because it is always eight inches or longer.

FREE Digital Copy, Updates, and More Information Available Here:
www.CashIsFun.com/cigar

Here is a list of common sizes, along with their approximate length and ring size. Ring size is measured in 1/64ths of an inch. Sizes will vary slight from brand to brand.

- Churchill   7"   48
- Torpedo   6.5"   52
- Corona   6.5"   44
- Pyramide   6.5"   44-52
- Toro   6"   50
- Perfecto   6"   47
- Panatella   6"   38
- Robusto   5"   50
- Petite   4"   30

#7
Choosing The Best Single

Wondering how to choose the perfect cigar? If you're a newcomer to the world of cigar smoking, here are a few tips to choosing the best cigar.

First, note the texture of the cigar. Squeeze it gently. Is very soft, or rigid? Ideally, the cigar should give slightly, but not too much. Very gently, squeeze the length of the cigar to check for lumps. A good cigar will have a consistent texture.

Next, inspect the cigar for flaws. Any cracks or discolorations are the signs of a lower quality cigar. The cigar's wrapper should be wrapped smoothly.

Finally, look at the ends of the cigar. Pay particular attention to the exposed end where cigar is lit. If you're new to cigars, it can be difficult to gauge the quality of the tobacco. The simplest way to judge the tobacco quality of a cigar is to inspect the color of the tobacco. If you note any abrupt color changes, this may indicate that the tobacco leaves were not laid out properly. Look for a cigar with a smooth blend of tobacco.

FREE Digital Copy, Updates, and More Information Available Here:
www.CashIsFun.com/cigar

#8
Top Brands

Try these top brands of premium cigars:
- Alex Bradley
- Arturo Fuente
- Ashton
- CAO
- Cohiba
- El Rey de Mundo
- H. Upmann
- Macanudo
- Montecristo
- Partagas
- Romeo y Julieta

#9
Types Of Cutters

- Straight - The single or double blade guillotine cutters are the most popular method of cutting cigars. If you're going to use this method, you'll want to go with a double blade because it will give a more even cut. Cigar scissors also fall into this category as well and provide a similar cutting action but some cigar experts think it is easier to get a straight cut with the scissors version.
- Wedge - V cutters let you slide a wedge into the cap at a specific depth instead of slicing the entire cap off this method is probably the most uncommon.
- Punch - The punch is a small sharp cylinder that lets you put a hole in the cap of the cigar. There is quite a mix of opinions on the punch method among cigar experts, some are strongly against using this method on a premium cigar, while others believe is it the best way to preserve and respect the skillfully rolled wrapper. These are often made onto keychains, and even if you prefer one of the other cutting methods, keeping one of these attached to

FREE Digital Copy, Updates, and More Information Available Here:
www.CashIsFun.com/cigar

your keys is a good backup method for any cigar enthusiast.

- Teeth - Of course, you can always just bite the cap off like Tony Soprano, but you're likely to damage the wrapper this way and cause it to unravel.

#10

Making The Perfect Cut

Although every cigar aficionado has their own proven method, here are some basic guidelines to get you started.

First, examine the head, or closed end, of the cigar. This is the part of the cigar that will need to be clipped. Determine where the 'cap' is. The cap refers to the part of the cigar where the tobacco leaf was used to close the cigar. Once you've found the cap, determine its length. As a general rule, you should not cut any further than the end of the cap. If you cut further than the cap, there's a good chance your cigar will unravel!

Use a good quality clipper to cut the head at the cap. You don't want a cheap cutter that will result in frayed or split cuts. You can purchase a special cigar cutter at your local tobacco shop that is designed to make clean cuts. Once you have your cutter, hold your cigar at eye level and make a fast and decisive cut just above the cap. Less is more when cutting—if you find your cut is too superficial, simply cut down a bit more.

FREE Digital Copy, Updates, and More Information Available Here:
www.CashIsFun.com/cigar

#11

Proper Lighting Technique

For new smokers, lighting a cigar can seem as daunting as learning to choose a good single. Here are four tips to guide you in lighting a cigar for the first time.

1. Use matches. If you must use a lighter, make sure it's butane lighter to avoid strong odors.

2. Warm the open end of the cigar (aka 'the foot' of the cigar) slowly over the flame, without touching it to the fire. Let a black ring form around the end.

3. Place the capped end of the cigar in your mouth and draw in slowly. Hold the cigar over the flame, about half an inch above it, again without touching. Continue to draw in until the cigar draws the flame. Turn the cigar slowly, spinning it to establish an even burn.

4. Once your cigar is lit, observe the burn you have established by blowing on it to light up the burning areas.

5. If the burn appears uneven, simply blow on the unlit sections to draw the burn, then take one or two draws from the cigar to establish an even burn.

FREE Digital Copy, Updates, and More Information Available Here:
www.CashIsFun.com/cigar

#12

All About Ashing

Unlike cigarettes, you do not ash cigars! Do not flick or tap or knock the ashes off your cigar. If possible, you should just let your cigar ashes fall off by themselves. A well made cigar should be able to support up to 2 inches of ash before falling. Leaving the ash on enhances the flavor of the smoke. If you are somewhere that you cannot just let the ash fall off by itself, such as your living room, then when the length of the ash gets close to an inch long, gently push the tip of the ash against the inside edge of your ashtray to break it off cleanly before going back to smoking.

Also, unlike regular cigarettes, cigars need their own special space to support their girth and ashes. Many cigar aficionados swear by the pleasures of finding the proper place to hold their cigars and ashes.

So what are the characteristics of a good ashtray? First of course, make sure the ashtray you buy is big enough to hold your cigars. Cigars come in varying sizes, so you will want an ashtray that can accommodate the single of your choice. Next, consider your personal style of smoking. Do you

FREE Digital Copy, Updates, and More Information Available Here:
www.CashIsFun.com/cigar

produce a lot of ash? Do you let your cigar rest for extended periods of time? These are all important considerations when choosing your ashtray.

Look for ashtrays made of metal, heavy glass, or ceramics. Ideally, you will want the ashtray to be big enough to hold the ashes for two cigars.

Where can you find the best ashtrays for your cigars? Many cigar aficionados swear by antique ashtrays. Search out flea markets and antique stores for good deals. Tobacco shops, mail order catalogues, and Internet shops are also good places to look.

#13

Being A Courteous Smoker

Smoking cigars may be a great source of pleasure in your life, but the courteous smoker knows that not everyone enjoys the taste (or smell!) of a good Cuban. With the fervor of anti-smoking campaigns in full swing, the importance of enjoying a good stogie while not offending others cannot be stressed enough. Simply remember that while you are smoking a cigar, it can be difficult to gauge the smell that others are experiencing. And don't forget that cigar smokes can leave a mighty strong residue on clothing, furniture, and even the walls! In order to enjoy your stogie without a heavy conscience, learn to become a considerate and courteous cigar smoker.

If you live with non-smokers, try to find a well-ventilated area of your residence where you can smoke comfortably. Although it may be tempting to lock yourself away in an office or bedroom, it's probably not a good idea to smoke in an enclosed area unless it has a window. Make sure you have easy access to the window. Never smoke in a closed area! You are more likely to inhale the toxic air from your own cigar. If possible, go outside to smoke. Pull up a lawn chair; relax on the porch, or

FREE Digital Copy, Updates, and More Information Available Here:
www.CashIsFun.com/cigar

any other open area where you can smoke comfortably. Get as far away as possible to non-smokers, especially children and the elderly. Remember that cigar smoke contains many carcinogens that can be easily inhaled by non-smokers.

If you must smoke a cigar away from your home, remember that the courteous and respectful smoker will only light up where legally permitted. Do no light up in a bar, hotel, or restaurant where smoking is clearly prohibited. The courteous cigar smoker will also make sure to smoke in the company of other smokers. If you are with someone who does not smoke, ask his or her permission. If they agree, be considerate about it. Make sure the smoke isn't wafting in their direction. Sit near an open window or space. Make sure the air conditioner or current is not moving the smoke in their direction! Also, make sure no one around you is eating. The secondhand smoke from a discourteous smoker is a surefire way to ruin a meal.

A courteous cigar smoker will also be aware of their ashes. If you must smoke outside your home, make certain to dispose of your ashes in a safe and appropriate container. Don't forget that ashes can easily blow away, especially in lower quality cigars. Don't litter with ashes, and be careful they don't blow near anyone around you.

#14

Quality Test

Now that you have some ash going, you can learn something about the quality of your cigar. Check the ashtray, the ashes left behind can speak volumes about the quality of your cigar. Here a few simple tips to determining the quality of your cigar...

First, note how fast your cigar burns. A cigar that seems to burn too quickly or disposes ashes that break apart easily is probably a lower quality cigar. If the ashes seem too messy, and doesn't break apart together, this may also indicate a lower quality cigar. Also, check the color of the ashes. If the ash color seems to change, the tobacco leaf mix may be of poorer quality.

The highest quality cigars, those that are well packed, will burn very slowly and burn stiff ash. The 'stiff ash' can remain intact up to two to three inches long, and remain on the cigar without breaking apart. A high quality cigar can be burned down to the nub.

#15

Pairing With Alcohol

Traditionally, the cigar has been paired with a strong drink. Popular spirits include rum, gin, brandy, and whiskey. Some argue that a good cigar should always be paired with a strong drink that has a hint of sweetness. Pairing cigars with beer is also becoming more popular as cigars become more main stream.

Experiment with different drinks to determine what best suits you.

Here are some suggestions:

- Scotch or Bourbon, neat or with 2 ice cubes; simple and flavorful, a nice match for any cigar, for scotch try Johnny Walker, or Glenlivet, for bourbon try Booker's, or Elijah Craig.
- Maker's Manhattan; classy all-American drink, a little sweet vermouth and a lot of bourbon.
- Extra Dry Bombay Sapphire Martini; gin, stirred and poured into a cocktail glass with a few olives, cold and refreshing.
- Rémy Martin; a good cognac or other type of brandy always goes well with a cigar.

FREE Digital Copy, Updates, and More Information Available Here:
www.CashIsFun.com/cigar

#16

Pairing With Food

Of course, you don't want to smoke while you are eating. But a cigar is always a good thing to enjoy after a great meal.

Here are some suggestions for great meals before lighting up your favorite cigar:

- A big medium rare ribeye steak with a baked potato.
- Grilled salmon on a bed of rice, with sautéd asparagus.
- Medium-rare bison burgers with hand made French fries.
- Lamb chops with mint jelly, and peppered green beans.
- Hot Italian Sausage with peppers and onions.
- A great filet and lobster tail, classic surf and turf, with grilled vegetables.

FREE Digital Copy, Updates, and More Information Available Here:
www.CashIsFun.com/cigar

#17

Get A Humidor

Humidors are used to store and protect cigars so that they are kept at their peak flavor. A humidor works by keeping a cigar at a constant level of humidity, ideally 70%.

The good humidor should close completely, with a tight fitting lid that will keep the cigars from the elements and prevent any exchange of moisture. Seams should be smooth and well fitted for cigars. Cedar, especially Spanish cedar, is ideal for the interior of the humidor.

Decent humidors can be purchased for $50 or less while the really nice, large capacity ones can be several hundred dollars. But remember that even if you only smoke a few cigars a month, a good humidor will save you time and money.

The markup on single cigars at your local tobacco shop or liquor store is quite high, and who wants to get in their car and drive to the store every time they feel like lighting up a good cigar? While if you have a humidor, you can buy bundles of higher quality cigars online for less per cigar and preserve them in your humidor at home indefinitely.

FREE Digital Copy, Updates, and More Information Available Here:
www.CashIsFun.com/cigar

#18

Vintage And Aged Cigars

Experienced cigar enthusiasts know the pleasures of a well-aged cigar. The subtle flavors and complex constitution of a well-aged cigar is indescribably and unforgettable. Like wine, many cigar aficionados swear by the process of aging. A great cigar, the argument goes, is an aged one. How can you attain a well-aged cigar that provides the mellow, complex flavors you crave? You can always fork over a good deal of your money and purchase a box of expensive vintage cigars. But you can always save the money and experiment with aging on your own...

First, know that you will have to be patient if you want a properly aged cigar. You will have to age your cigars for about a year in order to achieve the flavors and complex subtleties of a well-aged cigar. Also, know that in order to achieve the rewards of a well-aged cigar; you must begin the process with a high quality cigar. If you try to age a lower quality cigar, chances are any amount of aging won't improve their flavor significantly. In fact, almost all high quality cigars can be improved through the process of aging.

FREE Digital Copy, Updates, and More Information Available Here:
www.CashIsFun.com/cigar

#19

Don't Break The 70-70 Rule

To properly age, or even just store your cigars, environment is crucial. Cigars must be stored in a constant and stable environment. Follow the 70-70 rule. That means the humidity must be at a constant level of 70%, and the cigars must stay at a constant temperature of 70 degrees Fahrenheit. Any more and your cigars will get moldy; any less and the aging process begins to be stunted.

Maintaining a stable environment for your cigars is key; a constantly fluctuation environment can be disastrous. Swings in temperature and humidity cause cigars to expand and contract, cracking their wrappers and it may disrupt the aging process. Ideally, the space in the humidor should be about twice the volume of cigars. The lining should be cedar - cedar wood is highly aromatic wood, full of its own oils. With the passage of time, the interaction of the tobacco oils amongst themselves, and with the cedar oil of the wood it leads to a mellowing and blending of flavors resulting in that subtle complexity you can only get from proper aging.

#20

The Cuban Holy Grail

Every cigar aficionado knows that the very best cigars come from Cuba. Unfortunately, buying the best can often be a risky proposition. But many cigar enthusiasts are willing to take the risk to get a taste of the very best. If you're wondering just how one would get their hands on a box of Cubans, read on. Because of the relationship between the United States and Cuba, there are a lot of people looking to take advantage of cigar aficionados. Purchasing Cuban cigars should be done with great caution in order to avoid getting duped.

First, know that importing cigars from Cuba is considered illegal. The United States placed economic sanctions on the Cuban government in 1963. Ever since then, Cuban cigars have become the holy grail of cigar enthusiasts. There is, however, one loophole: visitors to Cuba who return from a sanctioned and licensed visit are allowed to bring back cigars. However, visitors are not able to bring back more than $100 worth of cigars, and they must be intended for personal use.

Any other ways of obtaining Cuban cigars is considered illegal. It is in fact illegal to buy, sell or trade Cuban cigars in the United States. Fines for illegal trading, buying or selling of Cuban cigars may face up to $55,000 in civil fines. This type of fine, however, is quite rare. The more likely scenario is that you'll have your cigars confiscated.

When purchasing a box of Cuban cigars, be prepared to fork over quite a bit of your cash. Prices can range from about $150 to $500 or more. If you're offered a box below these prices, chances are it may not be the real thing. Most Internet businesses that sell purportedly genuine Cuban cigars tend to be imitations. Always avoid shops or retailers that offer "discounted" Cuban cigars.

Some people get their hands on a box of authentic Cuban cigars by heading north to Canada. They buy them in Canada and repackage them so that they are not in their original Cuba packaging. They remove the rings and place the cigars in a different box. Customs agents tend to not inspect cigars carefully, and it is generally not considered a serious offense to bring Cuban cigars into the United States. In fact, many clerks at tobacco shops will even offer to repackage Cuban cigars for their customers.

FREE Digital Copy, Updates, and More Information Available Here:
www.CashIsFun.com/cigar

#21

Spotting Fake Cubans

If you have an opportunity to purchase a box of purported Cuban cigars, but have your doubts, take the time to examine the box before purchasing it.

Here are a few tips to help you spot the fakes... The most important thing to examine is the box. Authentic Cuban cigars will contain a green and white warranty seal on the left front side of the box. The seal will contain an insignia that has a picture of a shield and a hat. On the upper right hand corner of the box, you should find a white sticker that is placed diagonally with the word 'Habanos' printed on it. The overall appearance of the box should be neat and clean. If the box appears damaged, smudged, frayed, or marked, avoid it. If the color of the box is dull, don't buy it. Even if the cigars are the real things, their quality may have suffered in transport. Know that all authentic Cohiba's will contain the green and white warranty seal on the right hand side of the box.

On the bottom of the box of cigars, you should find a heat stamp with the words 'Habanos.' The heat stamp should be impressed onto the bottom of the box. Fake Cuban cigar boxes often find other ways

FREE Digital Copy, Updates, and More Information Available Here:
www.CashIsFun.com/cigar

to imprint this label, such as using rubber stamps or paper labels. You should also find a factory code stamp at the bottom that is stamped in green, blue or black ink. This stamp will tell you when and where the cigars were rolled.

If you can open the box, take the time to smell the tobacco. Cuban cigars will have a deep, rich aroma, unmistakable to dedicated cigar aficionados. If the smell is off, or very weak, chances are you do not have a box of authentic Cuban cigars in your hands. The cigars should be facing the same way, and the top row may appear slightly flattened. The caps on all the cigars should appear identical, and the foot of each cigar should be cut clean. The bands on all the cigars should also be identical, and should be arranged so that they face the same direction. If allowed, test the cigars out by pressing down on them. Feel along the entire length of each cigar, checking for soft or hard spots. The cigars should feel firm yet pliable.

#22
Give The Gift Of Smoke

Is there a cigar aficionado on your gift list? Wondering how to choose a decent cigar for a friend or loved one? Even if you know nothing about cigars or choosing a good cigar, just learning a few basics can help you sniff out (sometimes literally) a good cigar to give to a friend.

Fortunately, cigars have now entered the mainstream. Once the symbol of the rich and powerful, it's easier than ever for just about anyone to purchase a good cigar. Of course, you probably won't be able to buy your friend a box of top-tier Cuban cigars, but you can definitely buy them a good quality cigar that will put a smile on their face.

First, visit your local tobacconist or specialty smoke shop for the best quality and widest selection. Avoid 'drugstore' cigars. Although they may be inexpensive and convenient to purchase, drugstore cigars are usually filled with preservatives and generally of poorer quality. They may contain, at minimum, saltpeter, paper, glycerin, and other preservatives and irritants. You should make sure that the cigars you purchase are made of 100%

FREE Digital Copy, Updates, and More Information Available Here:
www.CashIsFun.com/cigar

tobacco. If you have any questions regarding the cigars ingredients, ask the salesperson. An experienced and knowledgeable sales clerk will be able to tell you extensive information about the ingredients.

Your local tobacco shop is a good place to shop because you will generally be allowed to smell and touch the cigars. Squeeze the cigar gently. A good quality cigar will give a little when squeezed. The cigar should be firm, with no excessively soft or hard spots. Never buy a lumpy cigar. Look at the wrapper. If you notice any drying or discoloration, best not to buy it. Ideally, the wrapper should be tight and smooth. Inspect the color of the tobacco to make sure it is even. Do this by inspecting the end of the cigar. Some color variation is normal, but if the color changes abruptly, chances are the cigar was not rolled properly. A cigar that is not rolled properly may result in an uneven burning and unpleasant odors.

If you're not sure how much your friend smokes, choose a longer cigar. Longer cigars tend to have a 'cooler' taste—an excellent choice for beginners. If you know your friend is an experienced and regular smoker, choose a cigar that is greater in diameter. These cigars tend to have a richer flavor that experienced smokers will appreciate.

FREE Digital Copy, Updates, and More Information Available Here:
www.CashIsFun.com/cigar

#23

Blowing Smoke Rings

Do you yearn to blow smoke rings with your cigar like a pro? Stogie aficionados often speak of the ceremony-like deliberateness of smoking a good cigar. Blowing smoke rings is the mark of a smoker who enjoys the smooth and relaxing effects of smoking. But how do you blow a good smoke ring? Some argue that it cannot be taught--that it will simply come to you with time and practice. Regardless, here are a few tips to get you going.

Veteran smokers note that in order to blow a good smoke ring, you will need to create dense smoke. Draw a deep, dense smoke puff into your mouth. Hold the smoke there and then open your mouth slowly and deliberately. Open your mouth, shaping your lips into a rounded 'O.' and pull your tongue back as you expel the smoke.

Keep in mind that you are not exhaling the smoke, but simply pushing it out of your mouth. Also keep in mind that this maneuver will not work if there is even a slight breeze in the air. Make sure you try it in a location with still calm air.

FREE Digital Copy, Updates, and More Information Available Here: www.CashIsFun.com/cigar

#24

Fighting The Beetles

Your cigar box may be at risk of a secret predator. Many cigar aficionados have been shocked and repulsed at finding their treasured cigars infested with Lasioderma Serricorne, also known as tobacco beetles. This dreaded beetle feeds on your precious cigars. They don't care if your cigars are drugstore mass-market brands, or imported beauties.

The tobacco beetle exits in all countries where tobacco is produced. It thrives on tobacco plants, infesting their leaves before it is processed. Tobacco beetles thrive in hot climates, and especially in the warm Caribbean countries where much of the world's cigar tobacco is produced. Tobacco beetles lay larvae that are white and up to 4 mm long. When the larvae hatch, they produce moths that proceed to hungrily eat their way through the tobacco leaves. Unfortunately, the tobacco beetle has been known to survive the process of fermentation and production that is used to make most cigars. Although many countries have made the effort to rid their tobacco crops of this dreaded pest, mostly by spraying crops with gases, the tobacco beetle has proven highly resistant.

FREE Digital Copy, Updates, and More Information Available Here:
www.CashIsFun.com/cigar

If the tobacco beetle survives into the finished product, many cigar enthusiasts may open their cigar boxes to find that their cigars have been eaten through. Sometimes the presence of the tobacco beetle can be detected through the presence of small puncture-like holes on the wrapper.

Your microwave may be your best defense in destroying the tobacco beetle larvae. Before using your microwave, remove and dispose of any infested cigar from your collection. The rest of your cigars can be treated. In order to rid the remaining of your collection of this pest, you should make sure to microwave your cigars together, never individually. Microwave them for about three minutes. After being warmed, immediately place the cigars into the freezer. After freezing them for 24 hours, remove them and allow them to thaw at room temperature. After they have thawed completely, place them in a humidor. This treatment has proven effective in removing the presence of the tobacco beetle. Before removing a cigar from the humidor to be smoked, examine each cigar individually. If the cigar shows no evidence of infestation, it is safe to smoke.

FREE Digital Copy, Updates, and More Information Available Here:
www.CashIsFun.com/cigar

#25

Cigar Bars

Cigar bars started to become popular in the mid-1990's when smoking bans were passed that provided exceptions for establishments that catered specifically to smokers.

These are often upscale establishments that allow clients a plush and comfortable smoking environment, sometimes with humidors that have special locks for individuals. Cigar bars also usually serve food and alcohol.

Cigar bars are an excellent place to smoke with your friends who share your interest in cigars, and interact with other smokers.

FREE Digital Copy, Updates, and More Information Available Here: **www.CashIsFun.com/cigar**

#26

Cigar-Friendly Activities

There are not many activities that you can participate in while smoking a cigar, however there are a few activities that are popular with cigar smokers.

Golfing and fishing are two activities often enjoyed by cigar smokers. They're always done outdoors so they provide a relatively friendly environment for cigar smokers away from the glares of non-smokers. Plus you can just let your ash fall anywhere, since it'll just land on the ground at the golf course (though make sure not to ash on the green), and on the boat pretty much every surface is made to be cleaned easily, so a little ash can be wiped off with no problem.

Many products, websites, and even specific cigars are made especially for people who like to enjoy a good cigar while enjoying a day of golfing or fishing.

Here's a few things to keep in mind while smoking during any outdoor activity:

- Those matches probably won't do the job if there's any wind. Be sure you have a good butane lighter with you so you won't have any problems.

- Get a good cigar case. Leather cigar cases that hold 2 or 3 cigars are important to keep your cigars protected while among your golf or fishing equipment. You can get a good case for anywhere from $15 to $100.
- Break out your favorite Churchill or other large cigar. You will have lots of time while you're waiting for the people in front of you on the course or waiting for that next largemouth bass to hit your line.
- Be sure you have a good place to set your cigar down. While you're taking your shot or fighting your big catch of the day, your cigar can sit and wait for you.
- Bring something good, but maybe not the best. Have a cigar you enjoy, but depending on your budget, keep in mind that you will be distracted with the activity at hand and won't be able to enjoy the cigar as much as if you were sitting on your porch with a glass of scotch.

#27

Parties

If you have a few friends who like cigars, passing some out at any party would be a hit, especially any "classy" event or while watching the big game. However, cigars go especially well with a bourbon tasting party. Here are some things to remember for having a good bourbon tasting party:

- Carefully choose a group of 5-8 good bourbons.
- Provide good cigars and make sure at least one good cutter and plenty of ash trays are available on the table.
- Play Frank Sinatra, jazz, or piano music.
- If you provide food, consider example ideas from Lesson #16 or appetizers such as caprese.
- Some people like to drink bourbon with ice or water, but for a bourbon tasting, sipping on the bourbon from a shot class or maybe a cordial glass is best.
- As you try each bottle, inform your guests about the price, proof, and history of each brand. Encourage your guests to talk about the flavors they taste in each.

Coming Soon:
CashIsFun.com

CashIsFun.com is a new site coming soon with practical information about all the fun, exciting, ridicules, and interesting things you can do with a little cash.

Point your browser to the page below to sign up for site updates, a free PDF copy and mp3 audiobook copy (when it becomes available), a great directory of cigar related sites, and other info... all for free!

www.CashIsFun.com/cigar

Did you enjoy this book?
Loan it to a friend or buy a copy for them.
Makes a great gift! And smoking with a good friend always makes the experience even better.

FREE Digital Copy, Updates, and More Information Available Here:
www.CashIsFun.com/cigar

Health Risks

Before we get started, here are some things you should know about cigar smoking and your health...

We have all heard about the dangers of inhaling second hand smoke. Many people wonder if the dangers of inhaling cigar smoke are just as bad, or more. Unfortunately, it appears that being exposed to secondhand smoke from a lit cigar can be just as dangerous, if not more dangerous, than regular cigarette smoke.

All secondhand smoke emitted by tobacco products are classified as environmental tobacco smoke. Environmental tobacco smoke refers to all the secondhand smoke released from tobacco products that are lit, such as cigars or cigarettes. Research indicates that the smoke from cigars and cigarettes releases many of the same types of irritants. Both cigar and cigarette environmental tobacco smoke contain nicotine, carbon monoxide, hydrogen cyanide, and ammonia. The environmental tobacco smoke from cigars and cigarettes also releases well-known carcinogens such as vinyl chloride, benzene, arsenic, hydrocarbons, and nitrosamines. Cigars, because of their size, usually release more environmental tobacco smoke than cigarettes. Being around cigar smoke, then, can pose more of a health threat than inhaling secondhand smoke from a lit cigarette.

Even though both cigars and cigarettes release similarly toxic environmental tobacco smoke, there are some key differences between the two. These differences are related to the very different ways

FREE Digital Copy, Updates, and More Information Available Here:
www.CashIsFun.com/cigar

that cigars and cigarettes are manufactured. The production of cigars consists of a long process of fermentation and aging. During the production and fermentation process, large amounts of carcinogens are produced. Once a cigar has been fermented and aged, they are wrapped in a nonporous wrapper that keeps the cigar from burning too quickly. The fermentation process and nonporous wrapper both contribute to the high concentrations of carcinogens in the smoke of a lit cigar. When a cigar is lit, the carcinogenic compounds produced during the fermentation process are released. The nonporous wrapper also contributes to an unclean burn that is high in carcinogens.

More info here:

http://www.cancer.gov/cancertopics/factsheet/Tobacco/cigars

Cigar Sites Directory

Here are some of the best cigar sites out there, however you can get an even more thorough list by signing up at *www.CashIsFun.com/cigar*:

- **AbsoluteCigars.com** - Full range of fine Havana cigars delivered worldwide from Switzerland.
- **ACigarSmoker.com** - Thorough cigar reviews and information.
- **AlecBradley.com** - Great premium cigar brand.
- **BirminghamCigars.com** - Birmingham, AL and online smoke shop.
- **CheapHumidors.com** - Retail site specializing in humidors, but selling cigars too.
- **Cigar.com** - Pretty obvious. Retail site with lots of different sampler pack options.
- **CigarAficionado.com** - The website for the magazine of the same name, lots of good cigar information here.
- **CigarAsylum.com** - Good cigar forum.
- **CigarAuctioneer.com** - An auction site just for cigars and related items.
- **CigarBlog.net** - Cigar news and review site.
- **CigarInspector.com** - Regular, illustrated and detailed reviews of both Cuban and non-Cuban cigars.
- **CigarJack.net** - Cigar news and review site.

FREE Digital Copy, Updates, and More Information Available Here:
www.CashIsFun.com/cigar

- **CigarPass.com** - Active cigar forum where you can talk with other cigar smokers.
- **CigarPlaces.com** - An interactive map that allows cigar lovers to find cigar bars and cigar friendly restaurants.
- **CigarsDirect.com** - Retail site a wide variety of premium cigars and accessories for sale.
- **CigarSecrets.com** - Solid cigar Information for every level of smoker.
- **CigarsInternational.com** - Big retail site with a good cigar of the month club.
- **CigarSmokers.com** - Good cigar forum.
- **CoastalCigars.com** - Cigar gift packages and cigar tastings/rollings for special events.
- **CubanCigarWebsite.com** - Great source of information about post-revolution period Cuban cigars.
- **Famous-Smoke.com** - Large retail site of a Pennsylvania smoke shop that's been around since 1939.
- **Humidor.com** - Also fairly obvious. A retail site with humidors, lighters, and cutters.
- **HumidorVault.com** - Retail site selling many different kinds of humidors.
- **JRCigars.com** - Claiming to be the world's largest cigar store, JR is a retail site with lots of cigars and cigar related equipment.

- **KinkyCigars.com** - Premium cigar brand from singer, songwriter, novelist, humorist, and politician Kinky Friedman.
- **LittleCigarFactory.com** - Small cigar company, "The Highest Quality In Hand rolled Cigars."
- **MDCigars.com** - "The Best Little Cigar Store on the Net!"
- **MercerCigars.com** - Merida, Mexico and online smoke shop.
- **MikesCigars.com** - Large retail site of a Florida smoke shop that's been around since 1950.
- **NashvilleCigarClub.com** - Site for cigar smokers in Nashville; get a discount at local cigar shops.
- **OldHavanaCigar.com** - "A Taste of the Good Life" a place for premium hand rolled cigars and accessories at reasonable prices.
- **Puff.com** - Cigar news and forum site.
- **SautterCigars.com** - Smoke shop of London with excellent online selection of cigar-related items.
- **StogieChat.com** - Great cigar forum.
- **StogieGuys.com** - A great blog site with reviews and articles about cigar smoking, great site to visit daily.
- **StogieReview.com** - Great review site for cigar and cigar related items.
- **TomsCigars.com** - Very good cigar blog and review site.

FREE Digital Copy, Updates, and More Information Available Here:
www.CashIsFun.com/cigar

Notes

FREE Digital Copy, Updates, and More Information Available Here:
www.CashIsFun.com/cigar

FREE Digital Copy, Updates, and More Information Available Here:
www.CashIsFun.com/cigar

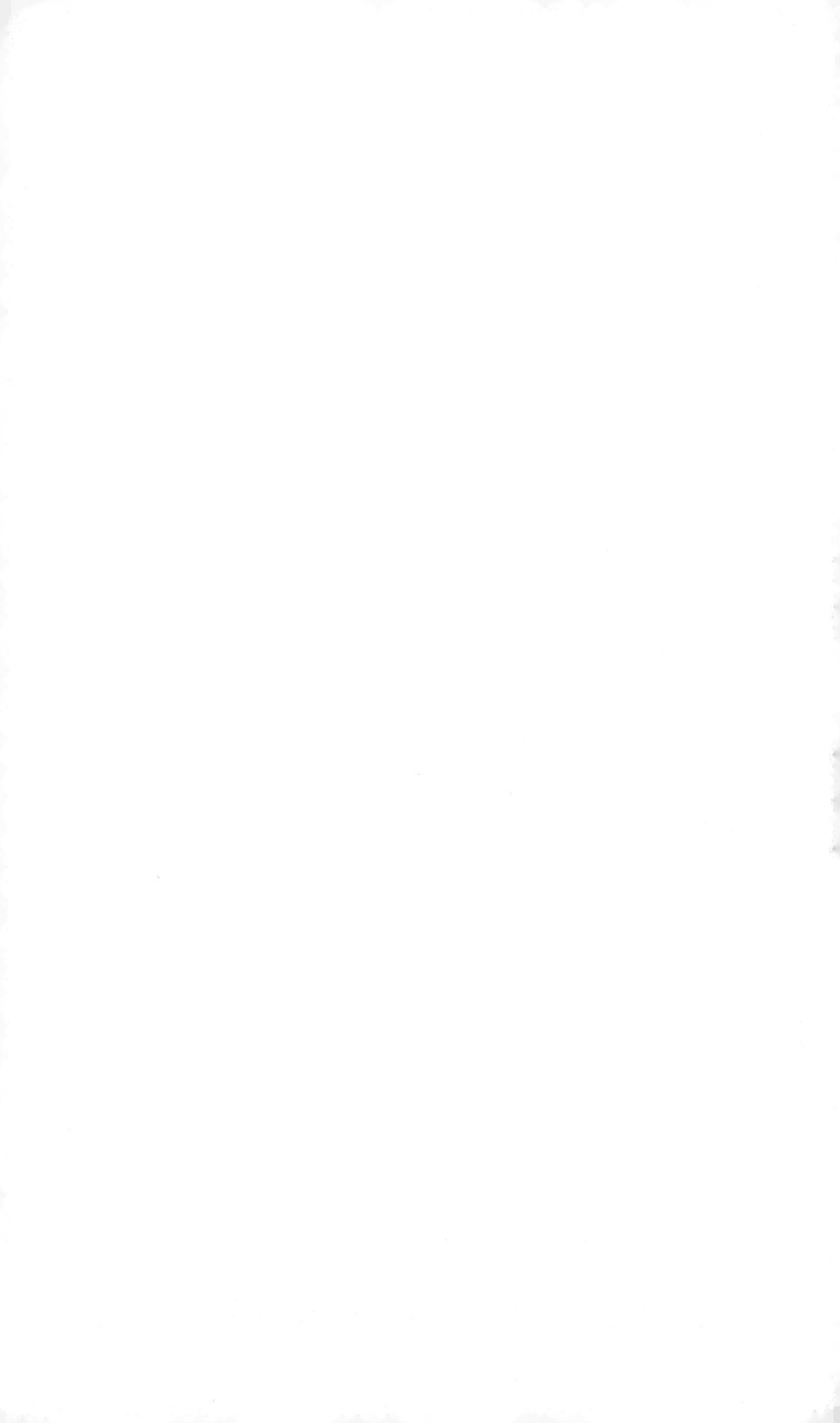

Made in the USA
Lexington, KY
17 August 2011